YOGA MAMA

18 Easy Yoga Poses
for Expectant Mothers

PATRICIA BACALL

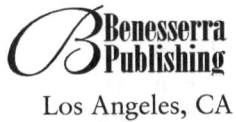
Benesserra
Publishing
Los Angeles, CA

Benesserra Publishing
Los Angeles, CA 90025
800-931-7007
First Edition
Print ISBN: 978-15142669-8-4
Ebook ISBN: 978-0-9863577-1-8

Disclaimer

Although the author and publisher have made every effort to ensure that the information in this book was correct at press time, they do not assume and hereby disclaim any liability to any party for any injury, loss, damage, or disruption caused by errors or omissions, whether such errors or omissions result from negligence, accident, or any other cause.

Patricia Bacall and Benesserra Publishing specifically disclaim liability for incidental or consequential damages and assume no responsibility or liability for any loss or damage suffered by any person as a result of the use or misuse of any of the information or content contained herein, and assume or undertake no liability for any loss or damage suffered as a result of the use or misuse of any information or content or any reliance thereon.

The purpose of this book is that of education and entertainment, and it is not intended as a substitute for the advice and guidance of a qualified yoga teacher or the medical advice of physicians. The reader should regularly consult a physician in matters relating to his/her health, particularly with respect to any symptoms that may require diagnosis or medical attention. Always consult your physician before beginning any exercise program. This general information is not intended to diagnose any medical condition or to replace your healthcare professional. Consult with your healthcare professional to design an appropriate exercise prescription. Always work within your own range of limits and abilities. If you have any medical concerns, talk with your doctor before practicing yoga. If you experience any pain or difficulty with these exercises, stop and consult your healthcare provider. Common sense and caution should be used when embarking on any physically demanding endeavor.

Table of Contents

CHAPTER 1

Prenatal Yoga—
Importance and Benefits

You've probably heard yoga is good for both mind and body. And you probably know it involves poses, breathing, and meditation. But what you might not know is that yoga leads to improved health, vitality, and well-being using specifically defined physical movements, mental exercises, and breath. Nearly 80 percent of people who practice yoga say they do it to increase their flexibility. Something else you might not know—you can do yoga while pregnant. It's called prenatal yoga. Yoga is all about becoming more in tune with your body—and what could be a better time to connect with your body than when there's a new life growing inside you?

What It Is

Prenatal yoga is a yoga practice specifically designed for pregnant women. It focuses on two main goals. The first is to help alleviate the aches and pains you're likely to experience during pregnancy. The second is to stretch your body, to make adequate room for your growing baby. And there's another benefit: some of the same poses and breathing techniques you use to alleviate aches and pains during pregnancy can end up being just as effective during labor.

Why a Regular Yoga Practice Won't Cut It

Although prenatal yoga may feature some of the same poses you'd find in any regular yoga practice, you're not always going to perform the poses in exactly the same way. It can be tough to stay balanced, sometimes even to stay upright, while leaning and stretching while pregnant. But prenatal yoga takes your body's changes into account, making adaptations to existing poses and introducing new ones, helping you to safely and effectively perform a regular yoga practice.

While prenatal yoga will have a major focus on stretching and restorative poses, don't expect to simply be lying on your mat the whole time. You'll be breathing, moving, stretching, bending, and grooving. Just how much you do so largely depends on where you are with your non-prenatal yoga practice, however. If you have a regular yoga practice and are more experienced, you can ease into a prenatal practice by paying attention to the poses you're already doing. If you're just starting to practice yoga, go slowly, and be open to your body and practice changing on a weekly basis. Your routine also depends on where you are in your pregnancy.

FIRST TRIMESTER TIPS

Even those experienced at yoga might not notice much difference between a regular yoga practice and a prenatal one yet. But there are differences. In the first

2

trimester there won't be many restrictions on the types of poses you can perform at this stage, but you want to stay keenly aware of how you're feeling, paying attention to the major changes occurring in your endocrine and other bodily systems. Your body will tell you if you're going too hard, too long, or practicing poses you'd be better off modifying or avoiding. And pay extra attention to hydration levels—your body needs a little more water when you're pregnant, even this early on.

SECOND TRIMESTER TIPS

The hormones that loosen your joints should be out in full force during your second trimester, and your center of balance will be different. Move carefully. Move gently and slowly, without holding any single pose for an extended period of time. And skip any poses that leave you lying flat on your back, as you want to keep a constant blood flow to your uterus.

THIRD TRIMESTER TIPS

Welcome to the world of walls and props. Both will be extremely helpful during this stage of your prenatal yoga practice. Walls and chairs are ideal ways to support yourself in standing poses. Blocks, straps and other props can help to maintain stability. Avoid holding any single pose for an extended period. Your goal is to keep moving, regardless of how slow that movement needs to be.

Benefits of Yoga during Pregnancy

You've already gotten a sneak peek at a few of prenatal yoga's benefits earlier in this chapter, but they're definitely worth restating. We've added them to our master list outlining what a regular prenatal yoga practice can do for you.

- **Alleviates pregnancy pains:** Pregnancy brings new aches and pains to your body; yoga gives you the tools you need to alleviate them. Certain poses can target specific areas that need attention, while restorative poses with generous props can help you slip into restful bliss.

- **Stretches your body to make room for growing baby:** Your baby will thank you for the extra elbow, knee, and foot-kicking room you give him or her with your regular practice. Again, specific areas can be targeted.

- **Decreases pain and discomfort during labor.** Some of the same poses that sooth your body, mind and soul during pregnancy can do the same when you're in labor. Your body's increased flexibility and suppleness can also make delivery easier.

- **Helps you cope with physical and emotional changes.** Pregnancy brings dramatic changes to your body and mind. Yoga not only makes you more aware of and in tune with these changes, it also gives you the tools you need to stay centered and serene while they're taking place.

- **Builds endurance:** Yoga can boost your stamina on three different levels—physical, mental and physiological. Yoga breathing techniques also teach you how to make the best use of your oxygen, delivering it to the muscles that need it most.

- **Perks up posture.** Pregnancy can do a number on your posture. Yoga helps to strengthen the shoulders and back, two important factors in proper posture. Many poses are also known for opening up the chest, which can instinctively prompt you to stand up tall.

- **Teaches you to relax, and deal with stress.** One branch of your nervous system controls your internal organs, and it has two parts—the sympathetic and the parasympathetic. The former kicks in when you're stressed, prompting the "fight or flight" response. The latter controls daily functions, gracing you with the "rest and digest" state. Yoga prompts the "rest and digest" state through controlled breathing and slow movements. It calms your body, and through it, your mind. Breathing while moving through the poses also helps you breathe more deeply.

- **Include breath work and meditation for even more soothing effects.** Combining yoga's breathing techniques with meditation helps you focus, blocking out the white noise of your thoughts. This is a prime way to eliminate stress.

With so many benefits, prenatal yoga is a wise move for both you and your baby. You're both likely to have a calmer, less stressed, more comfortable pregnancy.

CHAPTER 2

What Pregnancy Does to Your Mind and Body

Pregnancy can give be a wild ride—of hormones. The physical changes will be obvious to everyone around you, but on you'll also be going through a list of hormonal and emotional changes that can charge you up, bring you down, and swing you everywhere in between. But the joy you feel when you finally bring a new life into the world will likely outweigh any lows.

HORMONAL CHANGES

There are six key hormones that affect you during your pregnancy, and they will cause some of the biggest changes you'll experience. Here's the lowdown on what they are, and what they do.

HCG: Human Chorionic Gonadotropin

HGC is created by your uterine lining—the part of your body which eventually becomes the placenta. This hormone is what causes your body to prepare for the baby, which includes stopping your menstruation cycle. Your body's levels of this hormone skyrocket during the first 10 weeks of pregnancy, doubling as quickly as every two days. Although the cause of morning sickness is not definitively known, some doctors attribute it to rising HCG levels.

Progesterone

For the first 10 weeks of pregnancy, a temporary structure in the ovary known as the corpus luteum produces this hormone. Afterward, the placenta takes over. Like HCG, you'll get massive doses of progesterone early on in your pregnancy, and then levels plateau. It ensures your body will not reject the fetus' foreign DNA; it's also responsible for relaxing all the smooth muscles in your body—including those that form your uterus.

Because of this, progesterone can cause low blood pressure, dizziness, and fatigue, along with the array of gastrointestinal symptoms that can accompany pregnancy. These include belching, heartburn, nausea, vomiting, gas, acid reflux and constipation. Hair growth on your breasts and other unusual areas can also be attributed to progesterone.

Estrogen

Estrogen, like progesterone, is created by the corpus luteum until the placenta takes the over. Estrogen is essential to the development of the fetus, as well as the enhancement of the uterus during pregnancy. It too starts off strong, and then levels off over time. This hormone can be to blame for nausea, spider veins and an increase in appetite. It's also behind changes in the skin, both good and bad, from variations in skin pigmentation to that well-known pregnancy glow.

Oxytocin

Also known as the "love hormone," oxytocin has been shown to have an impact on bonding, trust, relaxation, psychological stability and motherly care. This is the one responsible for the blissful highs you might feel during pregnancy. It also plays a role in expanding the cervix, and prompts the nipples to produce milk.

Prolactin

This hormone also produces milk, but in a different way. Prolactin prompts breast tissue to begin lactation, and directs the milk's release. It gets up to 20 times its normal levels during pregnancy, which is good, since it can also have a soothing effect.

Relaxin

Relaxin is thought to help relax the uterine muscle, as well as the ligaments holding the pelvic bones in place. This hormone can increase up to 10 times normal levels during pregnancy. Its aim is to prepare the birth canal for delivery, but although it does a great job loosening the pelvic tendons, it also loosens up all the other ligaments in your body. This can result in aches, pain, and inflammation in your knees, hips, ankles and shoulders.

EMOTIONAL CHANGES

Are you ready for dramatic mood swings? No one ever is. But they'll be coming your way during pregnancy. The flood of hormones is to blame for the super-duper highs, the rock-bottom lows, and all other stages of your newfound emotional seesaw. You may also find yourself zapped of energy or extremely fatigued, another byproduct of hormones.

PHYSICAL CHANGES

You're going to gain weight. That much is obvious. But just how much depends on several factors, including your pre-pregnancy weight, your height, and how many new lives you're carrying. If you're at a healthy weight before your pregnancy, and are having only one child, the Institute of Medicine guidelines put your recommended weight gain between 25 and 35 pounds.

Other physical changes can include:

- **Breasts:** Your breasts generally increase in size and sensitivity, and your nipples darken. By week 12 to 14, your breasts may begin secreting colostrum, which is a mixture of water, minerals, antibodies and proteins that serves to feed your baby before your milk begins its regular flow.

- **Back:** The change in your posture, and the extra weight, can result in back pain.

- **Legs:** Your legs and their veins can become swollen, resulting in cramps and varicose veins. Your growing uterus can put pressure on the nerves in your legs, causing numbness and tingling.

- **Hands and fingers:** Numbness and tingling can also show up in your hands and fingers, usually first thing in the morning.

- **Lower abdomen and groin:** Hemorrhoids are unfortunately common during pregnancy, especially during the third trimester. They're caused by the weight of your uterus pressing on veins in your rectum. The frequent need to urinate is also common, thanks to the increased pressure on your bladder. You may also experience vaginal discharge, due to the increased blood supply to vaginal tissue.

- **Digestive system:** As you learned in the hormone section, digestive issues and pregnancy often travel hand in hand. Issues can range from constipation to heartburn, because your digestive system naturally slows during pregnancy, and your gastro-intestinal muscles relax.

- **Hair and nails:** The texture and growth patterns of your hair and nails may change during pregnancy, as a side effect of the hormonal changes.

- **Blood sugar levels:** High blood sugar levels can become a hazard, resulting in an ongoing condition known as gestational diabetes. A glucose screening is recommended between weeks 24 and 28 of pregnancy.

Other Changes

A handful of other changes may affect you during pregnancy, including:

- Morning sickness

- Headaches

- Trouble sleeping

- Stretch marks, which start off dark but lighten after birth

- Nose bleeds, or bleeding gums

Because every woman's biology is unique, you're likely to have your own unique combination of symptoms. But these symptoms often include a hormonal high, a bliss that you can enhance with a regular prenatal yoga practice.

CHAPTER 3

Importance of Breath

You spend most of your life breathing, and not thinking about it. But when you *do* think about it, amazing things can happen. The focused breathing used in yoga—known as *pranayama*—is an essential part of an effective yoga practice. In fact, some say the breathing is more important than the poses! This technique is particularly useful during prenatal yoga.

PRANAYAMA EXPLAINED

The term *pranayama* is the combination of *prana*, which means life force, and *ayama*, which means to draw out or extend. Put the two together and you end up with the translation: 'extending your life force.'

Ancient yogis believed each person was allowed a certain number of breaths to use throughout his or her life. If that's the case, then controlling your breath to make each breath more powerful and extended makes perfect sense. And even if it isn't true (the jury's still out), it makes sense to focus on your breathing, since to do so gives you power during pregnancy and beyond.

Pranayama for Prenatal Yoga

Pranayama and prenatal yoga are a perfect match. Controlled breathing allows you to feel your breath moving through you, and if you use a gentle, deep breath, pulling it up from your diaphragm, it loosens up your entire body.

Controlled breathing can also decrease stress hormones while increasing relaxation, particularly if you visualize your energy and oxygen moving through your body, to your baby with each inhale, your pelvic floor muscles softening with each exhale.

Breathing is the foundation of every pose in prenatal yoga. Learn to use it to your advantage during your practice, and you can use it just as effectively during the rest of your pregnancy. It can help you feel calmer, more centered, and more aware of your body, the world around you—and the baby growing inside you.

It can also—and this should come as no surprise— help during labor. It gives you something other than pain to focus on, and actually increase the strength in your muscles by increasing oxygen flow.

BAD BREATHING HABITS

Your breathing varies wildly when you don't pay attention to it, changing according to your mood, your temperature, or even what you had for lunch. Often, it's quite shallow, without using the power of the diaphragm. You're also unlikely to be giving your body and your baby the full extent of oxygen you could use, leaving you with a lineup of detriments.

These can include:

- Loss of part of your lung functioning, since the lungs aren't getting enough daily exercise. (Most people only use about one-tenth of their lung capacity.)

- A buildup of toxins in body cells due to inadequate oxygen intake, and inadequate output of carbon dioxide

- Increased fatigue due to decreased oxygen in the blood, and reduced circulation

- Reduced vitality, premature aging and a weakened immune system

- Possible anxiety, stomachaches, gas, heart burn, muscle cramps, sleep disorders, chest pain, dizziness, vision problems and heart palpitations

Doing something as simple as deepening and evening out your breath can give your body much-needed oxygen, calming your mind at the same time—and that's something that will benefit you even after your baby is born.

Prenatal Yoga Breathing Tips

If you're new to yoga, or to *pranayama*, it can be helpful to work on your breathing techniques before you combine them with poses. One way to start is with *samavrtti pranayama*, a breathing exercise that matches the quality and duration of your inhalations with that of your exhalations.

Starting with Samavrtti

First, establish a quiet, comfortable location. Lie down on whichever side is more comfortable, placing a pillow or folded blanket under your head to support your neck. Place another alongside your legs. Then bend your top knee, placing your top leg on the bolster. Make sure your knee and ankle are level with your hip, and that your hips are square.

Once you're in place, all you have to do is relax. Close your eyes, let your body go still, your nerves quiet. Then take note of your natural breathing pattern. It's likely to be shallow and irregular. Without trying to change your breathing patterns, pay particular attention to the following:

- The speed of your breathing
- Any pauses between inhalations and exhalations
- Durations and quality of your inhalations and exhalations

Once you've noted what your breath is doing, gently and gradually ease it into a smooth, even rhythm, where the length and quality of the inhalations are the same as the length and quality of the exhalations. Remain in this position, paying particular attention to:

- The overall increased elasticity and receptiveness of your lungs to your breath
- Opening the less-used portions of your lungs and rib cage

- Breathing more evenly, consciously and fully
- The increased volume of your breath, which should come without being forced
- Keeping your belly soft and deep, letting the breath roll in and out naturally

Some prenatal yoga instructors suggest imagining your belly as the ocean, your chest as the shore, and your breath as a wave washing up and falling back in a gentle rhythm. Continue this for up to 10 minutes.

Moving to Ujjayi Pranayama

Ujjayi pranayama translates to 'victorious breath,' and it uses the same technique as *samavrtti*—with one difference. As you breathing, slightly close your epiglottis—that flexible flap at the end of the larynx in your throat—to give your breath a voice. Listen to it, then, and make it as smooth and even as you can. Try to keep the same pitch and tone during every inhalation and exhalation.

Once you've mastered your breathing while lying down, move to a seated position. Move to your hands and knees, placing a small pillow between your ankles. Sit back on the pillow, with your hands on your belly and your eyes closed. Lengthen your spine by settling your hips and lifting your head toward the ceiling. Practice the breathing techniques you've learned so far, then move on to the next section.

HAPPY BABY BREATHING

This type of breathing aims to mimic the deep, full, easy breathing happy babies naturally enjoy. It's soothes the nervous system, and boosts oxygen flow to the uterus. This kind of breathing can bring relief during pregnancy, labor and birth.

Take a seated position on your pillow and begin to breathe. Concentrate on the feeling of fullness you experience as your belly expands with each inhalation. Sink your belly softly back toward your spine with each exhalation, imagining your giving your baby a gentle hug. Continue the practice for up to 5 minutes.

The power of *pranayama* becomes even more obvious when you see how perfectly it aligns with the benefits of prenatal yoga.

CHAPTER 4

Priming Your Mind—Why Learning to Relax is a *Must* During Pregnancy

Stress is part of daily life, and you don't get a free pass because you're pregnant. In fact, pregnancy can often bring on additional stressors. Physical discomfort, hormonal changes and mood swings, worrying about the birth and after, and work-related issues can all bring on additional stress, and it can be harmful not only to your health, but to the well-being of your baby. The impact might fade soon after birth, or it could affect your child in their early years and even into adulthood.

WHY RELAXATION IS A *MUST* DURING PREGNANCY

Dozens of studies have been conducted on the effects of stress during pregnancy, with a results summary reported by Emory University School of Medicine. Excessive amounts of stress and anxiety during pregnancy has been linked to:

- Higher chances of a preterm birth or miscarriage
- Smaller birth length and weight
- Problems with temperament and fussiness
- Issues with attention spans and emotional reactions

- Behavioral issues
- Lower scores in mental development measures
- Emotional problems

Before you totally freak out, however, keep a few things in mind. Normal amounts of stress, such as the stress you experience when meeting a last-minute work deadline or being stuck in a traffic jam, are not likely to have any notable negative effects. In fact, some studies have shown that mild to moderate amounts of stress may actually be beneficial for the baby. It may help strengthen the immune system, enhance motor development, and prepare the baby for his or her own later stressors, such as birth.

Even larger amounts of stress can be fine, provided you have the right tools to handle it positively. And prenatal yoga gives you those tools—and more.

HOW YOGA HELPS YOU RELAX

The greatest benefit of prenatal yoga is its ability to help you to relax. It does this not by teaching you how to block out the stressors entirely, but by bringing you through it with a calm, balanced mind.

The Relaxation Response

The combination of poses and breathing you perform in prenatal yoga can bring comfort and release. That feeling in turn causes a relaxation response. A reduced heart rate, lower blood pressure, and a decrease in stress hormones—all because you've started breathing differently!

And the best part is, you can use the same techniques to relax at any time. It not only decreases stress levels, but prepares you to better deal with stress at other times, too, including during labor. Stress hormones and the adrenaline they cause actually help to manage pain, but that doesn't mean they're easy to handle, and the relaxation response triggered by yoga's controlled breathing can help you stay much calmer.

The Conscious Release

Another way yoga helps you relax is by giving you an increased awareness of your body, mind and soul. When you become more aware of your being, you're able to pinpoint where you're full of tension and stress. And then you can consciously release it. Become aware of it, accept it, then let it go. Training your awareness to consciously release tension during your yoga practice allows you to do the same during labor and birth. Become aware of it. Accept it. Then let it go.

Taking it to Daily Life

Yoga's power of relaxation can help during pregnancy and beyond, as you incorporate the relaxation techniques learned on the yoga mat into your daily life. Whenever you're feeling overwhelmed or stressed, take a moment to calm your body and mind through controlled breathing, closing your eye, and concentrating on your breath, imagining it moving through you. Pinpoint the specific issue that's causing you grief, and gently let it go, accepting the world as it comes to you.

The benefits of this relaxation technique emerge quickly. Soon you're sleeping more soundly, and feeling more cheerful during the day. Stress and anxiety levels decrease, and

Feelings of happiness and fulfillment increase. This enhanced sense of overall well-being will also lead to a calmer, more peaceful pregnancy.

CHAPTER 5

Easy Mama Yoga Safety Tips

Prenatal yoga is one of the safest forms of exercise during pregnancy, because it was designed specifically for pregnant women. You can make it even safer by following these simple guidelines.

The first is to get approval from your doctor before engaging in a prenatal yoga practice, or any type of exercise routine. The second is to make your practice a habit, as a regular routine is more beneficial, and easier on your body, than long stretches of immobility broken up by bursts of exercise. Third, follow

PRENATAL YOGA DOS AND DON'TS

- **Do stay hydrated.** Water is your new best friend. Try to drink at least eight ounces, sipping before, during, and after your session. Aim for one cup every 20 minutes of your workout, more if the weather is especially humid or hot.

- **Don't get overheated.** This means Bikram yoga is out, as is performing your routine in any environment that is overly warm or stuffy. This is especially crucial during your first trimester, when major organs are developing in your baby's body. If your core temperature increases to more than 102 degrees for longer than 10 minutes, it can put your baby at risk.

Pregnancy can make you feel warmer to begin with, thanks to your increased metabolic rate and blood flow. Add exercise to the mix, and you can end up real hot, real fast. If you start feeling nauseous, dizzy, or uncomfortably warm, take a quick break to cool down. Peel off extra clothing layers or head for a cool shower or air-conditioned room.

- **Do dress properly.** Yoga is known for its comfortable, loose clothing, which is exactly what you want for your prenatal exercise. Choose breathable fabrics, dress in layers you can quickly remove and choose a supportive maternity bra to don beneath your yoga top.

- **Don't hold poses for extended periods.** Standing immobile for an extended length of time can make blood pool in your legs, causing dizziness. It can also reduce the blood flow to your uterus. Keep moving by switching between poses with slow, graceful and fluid movements.

- **Do get up slowly.** Slow, graceful and fluid should be the mantra for all movement you do in prenatal yoga, especially when it comes to getting up off the floor. Getting up too quickly can cause dizziness and loss of balance. Remember that your center of gravity shifts as your belly grows.

- **Don't lie flat on your back.** Poses that place you flat on your back should be avoided once you enter your second trimester, or even earlier if they make you uncomfortable. Lying flat on your back exerts pressure on vena cava, which transports blood to your heart. This could end up reducing blood flow to your uterus and brain, resulting in nausea, dizziness and shortness of breath.

- Make any necessary adjustments to poses, such as placing a pillow under your right hip to avoid putting pressure on the vena cava. Or try lying on your side, instead of your back, with your top knee bent and propped on a pillow.

- **Don't lie on your stomach.** Any pose that put all your weight on your stomach, such as the cobra, locust and bow poses, should be avoided. If you are experienced in yoga, and want to do some kind of backbend, try the bridge or camel pose.

- **Do consume extra calories.** Even though yoga is not necessarily known for its high calorie burn, you want to make sure you eat enough to account for you, your baby and the extra calories exercise eats up. Your doctor can tell you how many extra calories you should consume, but the general recommended amount is at least 300 above your daily intake if you're at a healthy weight.

- **Do warm up and cool down.** A good way to warm up prior to your prenatal yoga routine is with a few gentle head rolls and stretches. Warming up gets your joints and muscles ready for the more strenuous positions to come.

Cooling down can consist of more gentle stretching and engaging in a comfortable, restorative pose in a relaxed state of meditation. This can help get your heart rate back to normal while letting you fully enjoy the peacefulness that comes with your workout.

POSES TO AVOID

Lying flat on your back is to be avoided, but it's not the only position you shouldn't take during pregnancy. Yoga Journal recommends steering clear of any poses that may be potentially dangerous to you or your baby, such as:

- Twist that put pressure on your abdomen
- Deep backbends
- Deep forward bends
- Poses that involve lying flat on your belly

Inversions may or may not be risky, depending on your experience and how you perform them. Some say inversions should be altogether eliminated during pregnancy, while others say they can be adapted to be performed safely if they've been a part of your regular routine until now.

Using a wall or chair as support during the shoulderstand pose, for example, can allow you to use the pose for great relief during pregnancy if you're already familiar with it. But again, your doctor should have final say on your use of inversions.

THE ART OF ADAPTATION

Changes in your body during pregnancy call for changes in positioning for some of the traditional yoga poses you may want to perform. Remember that hormone relaxin? It relaxes your ligaments and joints in preparation for childbirth, but also increases your risk of injury should you happen to fall. Some adaptations you can make include:

- Modifying twists to only move your rib cage, shoulders and upper back – not your abdomen

- Bending from your hips instead of your back to keep your spine properly curved

- Moving against a wall during seated positions so you can keep your spine straight while supporting your entire backbone, from tailbone to shoulders

- Using props to help maintain your balance as your center of gravity continues to shift

But the most important safety tip of all is to listen to your body. Don't overdo it. Pace yourself. Set realistic goals. Know and respect your limits. Use common sense and these helpful guidelines to keep you and your baby safe.

Chapter 6:

Getting Started with Easy Mama Yoga

Now that you have a good grasp on what prenatal yoga is all about, it's time to make your final preparations before you actually hit the mat.

EQUIPMENT

Sticky mat: Yoga sticky mats have a textured surface specially designed to prevent slipping. They come in various thicknesses, colors and designs. Pick one that is thick enough to serve as a comfortable barrier between you and the floor. If you end up with one that's too thin to practice on in comfort, use two mats, or fold it over to give you more cushioning.

Blanket: These serve as padding when you need a little help making certain poses more comfortable. The serape-style, Mexican blankets are ideal for yoga as they feature a dense, non-slippery texture, and come in smaller sizes for easy folding and bunching.

Blocks: These provide support and assistance with specific poses you may find tough to achieve. If you're having trouble touching your toes when you bend over, for instance, you can use a block to make up the distance between your hands and the floor. They're also useful for maintaining balance in poses that require deeper stretches, or a single hand placed on the mat. Blocks come in various sizes, materials and colors. A 9-inch foam block should do the trick.

Straps: Also known as yoga belts, straps can help you deepen a pose or stretch. If you're finding it tough to reach your toes during a seated stretch, you can bend your leg, loop the strap around your foot, and then extend your leg with your hands holding the strap, bending your body as much as you can.

Straps are typically made of cotton, and come in different lengths. A 6-inch strap is a good size for most, but go for an 8-inch to 10-inch strap if you're on the tall side. There are also a variety of closure mechanisms to choose from. D-ring closures are the easiest to adjust and re-adjust, while pinch-buckle closures offer more sturdy support once the strap is adjusted.

Comfy clothes: The top consideration for yoga clothes is that they allow you to move, so you're not stuck with constant readjustments. Cotton and Lycra are good choices for materials, since they are comfortable and stay close to your body.

Support is another must, especially for prenatal yoga. Choose a supportive sports bra, then top it off with a yoga tank top and yoga pants or shorts. The yoga clothing industry is already serving expectant mothers, so you should have no problem finding yoga outfits for every stage of your pregnancy.

YOGA BREATHING REVIEW

Our third chapter went over how breathing techniques can be used to enrich your body, mind and soul. Breathing is an integral part of yoga, and it's especially important as you're moving through your poses. As you move into each pose, inhale through your nose, filling your ribs, belly and upper chest with air. Then exhale fully, also through your nose, pulling in your belly to help push out the air for a full release.

WARM UP EXERCISES

Even though prenatal yoga is less strenuous than most other types of exercise, it still needs a gentle warm-up to get your blood flowing and body prepped for your upcoming routine. The previous chapter mentioned head rolls as an ideal warm-up exercise. They can be performed by doing three deep, slow rolls to the right, and then to the left, while in a seated position. Others include:

Neck stretch: These deep, gentle movements help stretch and warm up your neck.

- Sit on your mat in a cross-legged position.
- Exhale and slowly tilt your head to the right, stopping the tilt when you feel a deep stretch in your neck.
- Hold the position, taking three deep breaths.
- Return your head to center and repeat on other side. Repeat three times.

Shoulder roll: This move can be done in either a sitting or standing position. It helps open up your chest and back.

- Stretch your arms out to your sides, placing your fingers on your shoulders.

- Inhale, bringing your elbows in front of you and then lift them toward the ceiling.

- Exhale, returning to the starting position.

- Repeat three times in each direction, with your shoulders rolling back and again with your shoulders rolling forward.

Toe and foot stretch: This move helps stimulate circulation while loosening your calf muscles.

- Sit up straight with your knees bent and legs tucked beneath you.

- Press your toes and balls of your feet firmly against the mat. Repeat.

The last thing you need to remember before you begin your yoga practice is that it doesn't have to end when your pregnancy does. Continuing a regular yoga routine can help calm your mind, ease your body, and bring peace to your soul, during pregnancy and labor and for the rest of your life. Namaste!

CHAPTER 7:

The Yoga Mama
Easy Yoga Pose Sequence

In this chapter you'll learn a few basic poses you can use during pregnancy. Remember, it's important to listen to your body! Always play it safe, and avoiding postures that put too much strain on your body.

THINGS TO REMEMBER

For those accustomed to advanced yoga moves prior to pregnancy, remember that some positions must be modified while you're pregnant. Although many poses can still be performed easily, the pressure and severe twisting can cause problems with the placenta and the baby. Some poses to avoid include:

- Bridge (after the fourth month) and other deep backbends

- Camel

- Poses balancing on one leg later in pregnancy, unless you use a wall for support

- Upward Bow

- Poses that engage the abdominals tightly, such as Boat Pose

It's safer to reserve these poses until after you give birth.

SEATED OR STANDING DEEP BREATHING

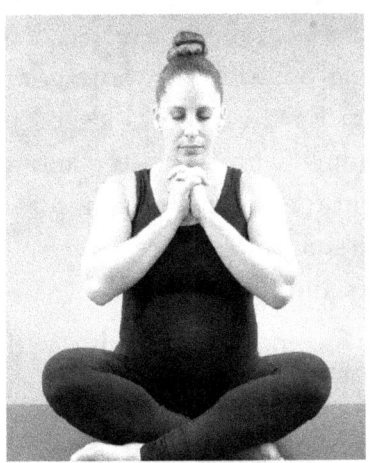

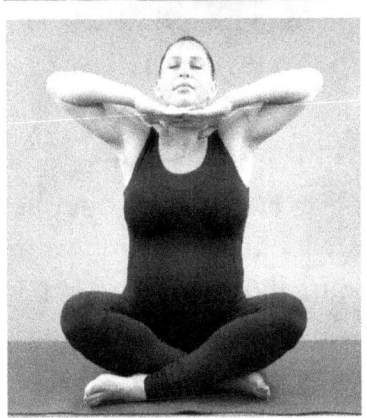

The seated or standing Deep Breathing exercise, also known as *pranayama*, delivers oxygen deep into the lungs to refresh and energize the mind and body. During the pose, the torso is lengthened and expanded, allowing oxygen to be delivered to the organs, muscles, and your baby so you can experience the renewing benefits.

How To Do It

This pose can be done in a seated or standing position, depending on which is more comfortable. You can sit on the floor in a cross-legged position, on a chair, or standing with your feet about hip distance apart with your toes facing straight forward. Whether sitting or standing, make sure your spine is straight, with shoulders and hips in line.

- Lace your fingers under the chin with your elbows pointing downward, and relax your shoulders.

- Inhale deeply, counting slowly to six, as you raise your elbows. You will feel the air expand your stomach, then your ribcage.

- Slowly start to exhale, counting slowly to six again. While exhaling, push your head back until you are looking upward toward the ceiling, bringing your elbows forward at the same time, until they are touching or close to touching, in front of your chest.

- Slowly begin inhaling, while bringing your head back down, and moving the elbows up again to the starting position.

- Continue for 10 sets on inhales and exhales.

- Never hold your breath; always be inhaling or exhaling.

Things to Remember

While doing this pose, the goal is to bring in as much oxygen as possible to experience the most benefit. If you begin to feel dizzy, stop doing the pose – you want to make sure you are providing the baby with plenty of oxygen, but not to the point that you feel faint.

As always, while there are many benefits for doing yoga while pregnant, you need to check with your doctor, and work with a professional to make sure that the proper modifications are used throughout your pregnancy for maximum safety and benefit.

SITTING OR KNEELING SIDE STRETCHES

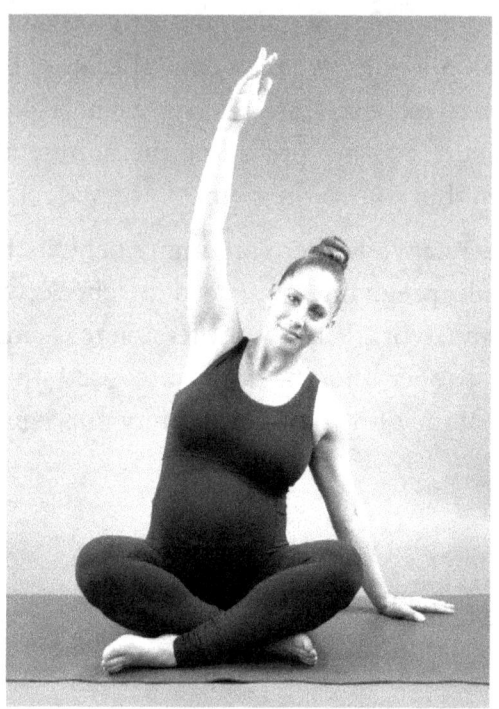

The sitting or kneeling side stretches open up the ribcage. During pregnancy, the spaces between the ribs often become compressed, making it difficult to breathe properly. By expanding these spaces, the chest is opened up, and the lungs can expand more freely.

How To Do It

This pose can be done sitting with the legs crossed, or by kneeling—whichever is most comfortable for you.

- Either sitting or from the kneeling position, put your right hand at your side on the floor with the palm down.

- Inhale slowly, pulling air deep into your lungs, feeling first your belly and then your chest expanding.

- While inhaling, raise your left arm so that it moves diagonally over your ear, reaching towards your right side.

- Make sure you are looking straight ahead throughout the pose, and that you are keeping your hips in the original position.

- Slowly exhale, moving back to the starting position.

Repeat this side stretch three to five times on the right side. With each stretch, try to stretch a little farther, but don't cause yourself pain or discomfort.

Switch your position so that your left hand is on the floor, and repeat the same steps, raising your right hand over your ear and towards your left side.

Things to Remember

While doing these stretches, make sure you are not allowing your shoulders to move up towards your ear when lifting your arm. You should also concentrate on keeping your hips centered and grounded as much as possible to make each stretch more effective.

Breathe deeply with each inhale, and exhale slowly – counting to six during both will help ensure you are drawing in a full breath, and exhaling it completely. If you don't feel your stomach and chest rising during the inhale, you're not breathing deeply enough.

CAT POSE TO NEUTRAL AND ROCKING CAT

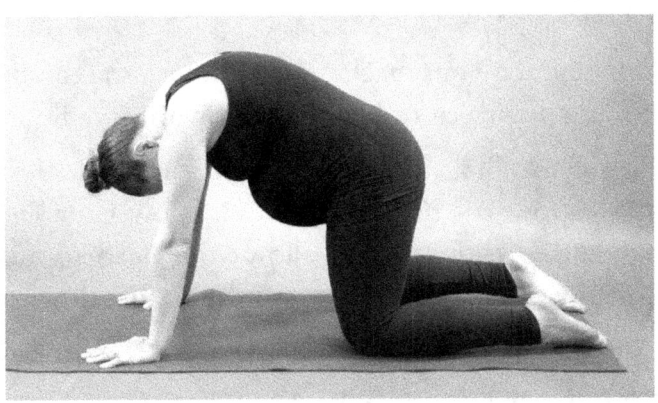

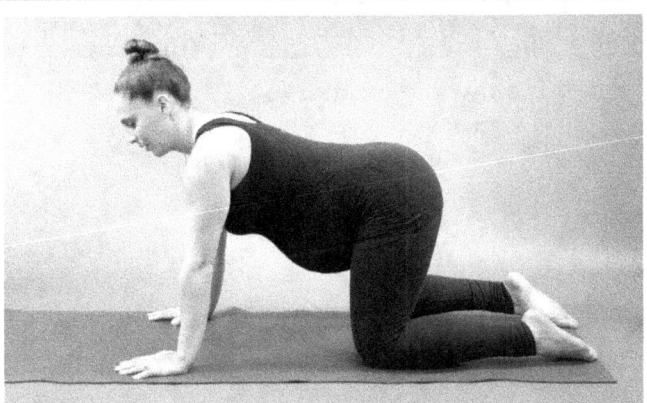

The Cat pose helps improve circulation, flexibility in the spine, and digestion. It also relaxes the mind and eases tension in the shoulders and upper back.

How To Do It

Start on all fours, ensuring that your hips are directly above your knees, and that your shoulders, elbows and wrists form a straight line perpendicular to the floor. Your head should be neutral, and neck in line with your spine, allowing you to look directly at the floor.

Make sure your back is in a long straight line, without allowing it to bow down towards the floor.

While exhaling, round your spine upward so that it moves towards the ceiling. Don't allow your knees or shoulders to move, but allow your head to move towards the floor without forcing your chin down.

Slowly inhale deeply, allowing your spine to move back to the neutral starting position.

Repeat five to ten times, making sure to keep your movements slow and steady.

THE ROCKING CAT

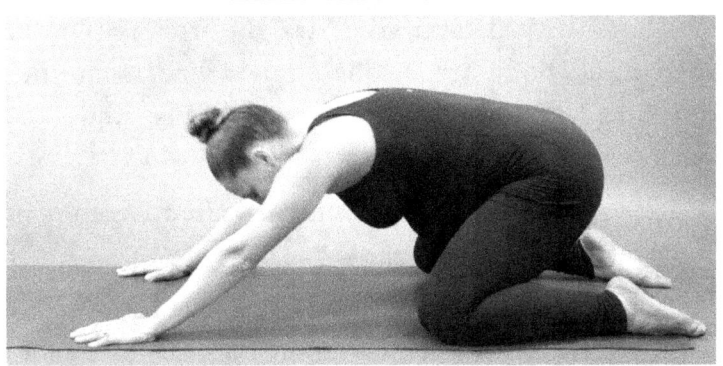

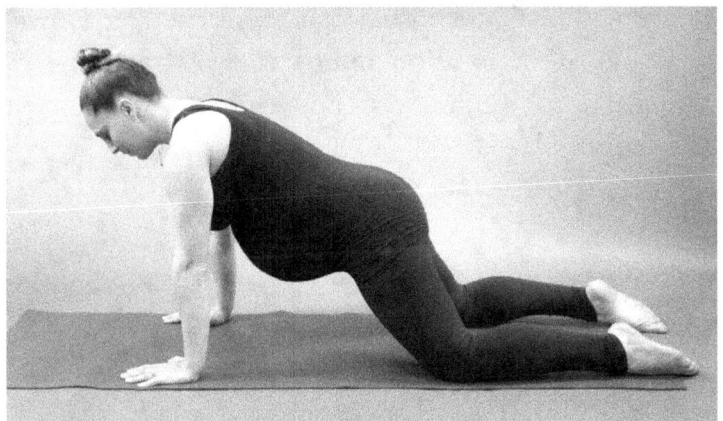

The Rocking Cat pose also helps relieve discomfort. You will move into this pose from the Cat.

In the neutral position, bring your toes together and tuck them under.

Push your hips back so that they are resting on your heels. At the same time, stretch your arms straight out in front of you.

You are moving into Child's pose, but make sure your

41

knees are wider than your belly to avoid compression.

Rock forward onto your straight arms until your thighs and body are in one straight line from your knees to your shoulders. Breathe deeply, and rock back onto your heels.

Repeat four to six times, making sure to keep your movements slow and steady.

When performing any yoga pose, make sure you are aware of what your body is telling you. If moving into the modified Child's pose is uncomfortable, slowly relax out of the position and try it again another day. You want to soothe your body, not make yourself uncomfortable.

CHILD'S POSE VARIATIONS FOR PREGNANCY

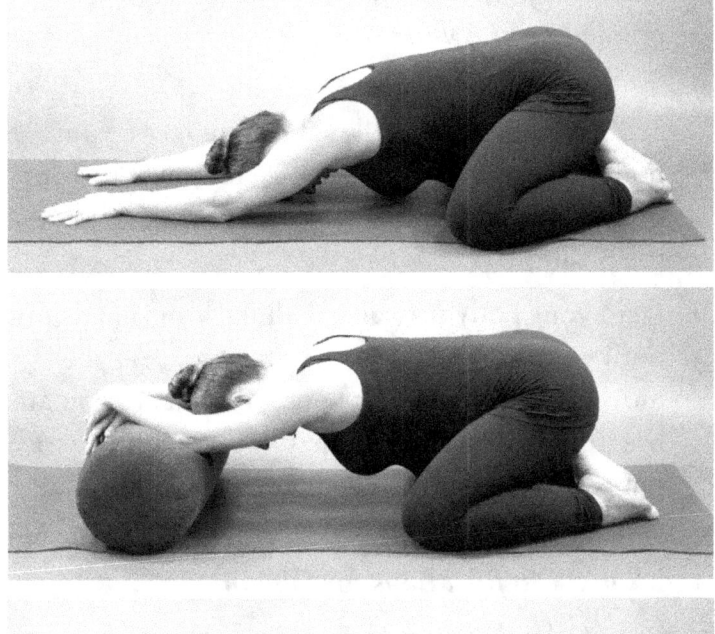

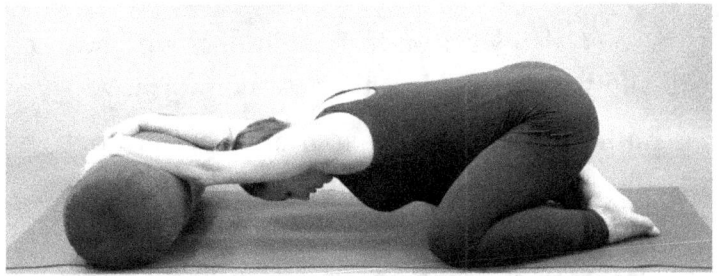

The Child's pose is both a spine lengthener and a hip opener. It's also used for relaxation, grounding, and for rest between poses. For pregnancy, this pose is modified to reduce abdomen compression.

How To Do It

- Start this pose by kneeling, with your toes pointed behind you.

- Your knees will be wider than hip width, to accommodate your belly when you move your body forward. You will be able to adjust to your own most comfortable width as you move into the position.

- Lean your body forward, walking your hands out until your arms are stretched forward. As you move your body into the pose, make sure you are breathing normally, and that you don't move too far – you should feel a gentle stretching through your arms, back, hips and shoulders.

Additional Modifications for Support

If you feel any discomfort, additional modifications will allow you to achieve the pose comfortably:

- Rather than stretching your arms out in front, fold them. Rest your head on top to make the stretch less intense.

- Place a thick blanket, towel, or pillow under your torso and between your legs.

- Roll up a towel to between your calves and butt for extra support.

Experiment with different modifications until you can hold the pose in a completely relaxed manner, without needing to engage any muscles to hold it.

When you come out of the Child's pose, make sure you use your arms to walk yourself back up into the starting position so that you don't have to strain or bring yourself out of the relaxed state that this pose provides.

COW POSE

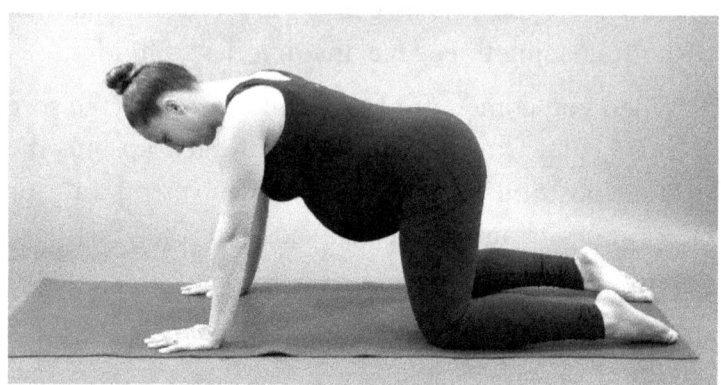

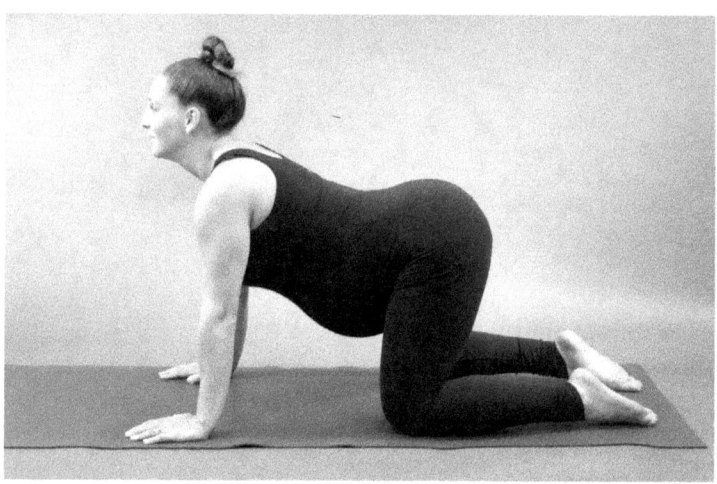

The Cow pose relieves back pain during pregnancy by releasing stiffness in the back and hips, strengthening the abdominal and pelvic floor muscles, and allowing the baby to move away from your spine for a little while. It's also beneficial during labor, especially for women experiencing intense back pain during labor—often caused by your baby's skull pressing against your lowed back. There's even evidence that this position can help when babies present with in breech birth prior to delivery. In some cases, holding the Cow pose for short periods has encouraged the baby to move into the correct head-down, backward facing position.

How To Do It

- Start the pose by getting into the 'tabletop', or all fours position, keeping your shoulders, elbows and wrists in line, and your knees directly beneath your hips. Make sure you are looking at the floor with your head in a neutral, centered position.

- Inhale slowly and deeply, lifting your chest and sitting bones so that they are moving towards the ceiling–your belly will lower towards the floor. At the same time, slowly lift your head so that you are looking straight ahead.

- Exhale slowly, moving your hips and chest back down into the neutral tabletop starting position.

Repeat the movement 5 to 10 times, focusing on breathing deeply, and feeling the stretch in your lower back and hips.

Things to Remember

This position is always useful, and can help immensely with lower back pain. But it's also great for opening the chest and hips. As long as you inhale and exhale completely when you're performing the pose, your oxygen levels increase—and that's good for you *and* your baby.

If you have any neck problems or injuries, keep your head in a neutral position rather than lifting it to avoid discomfort.

COW FACE POSE

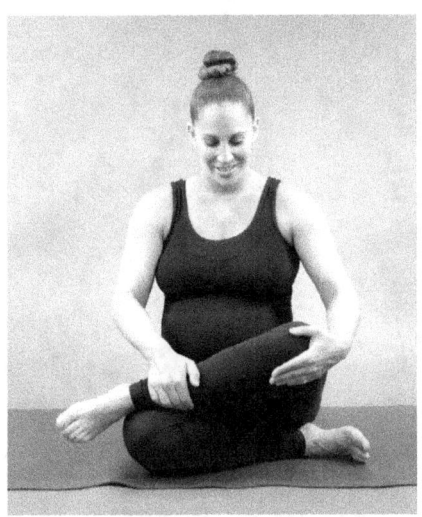

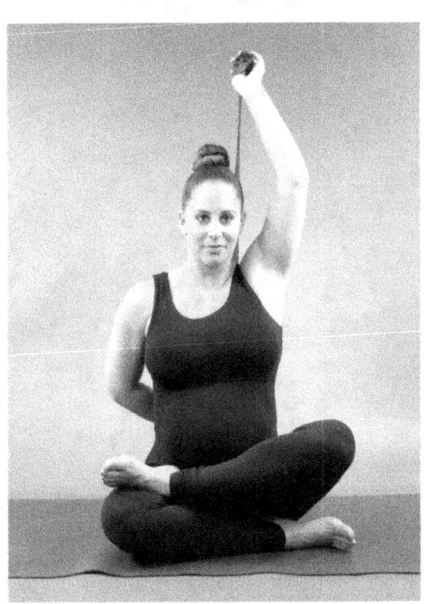

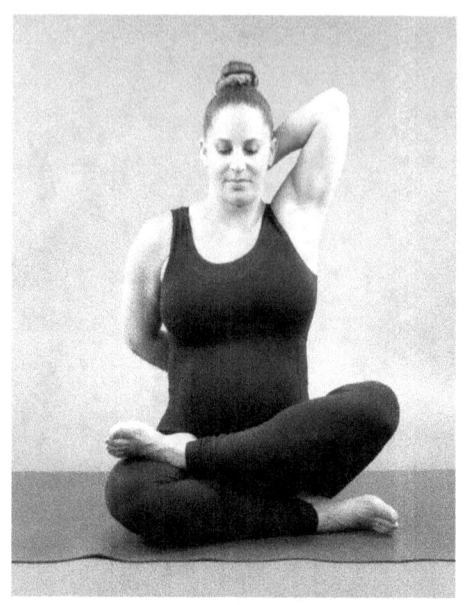

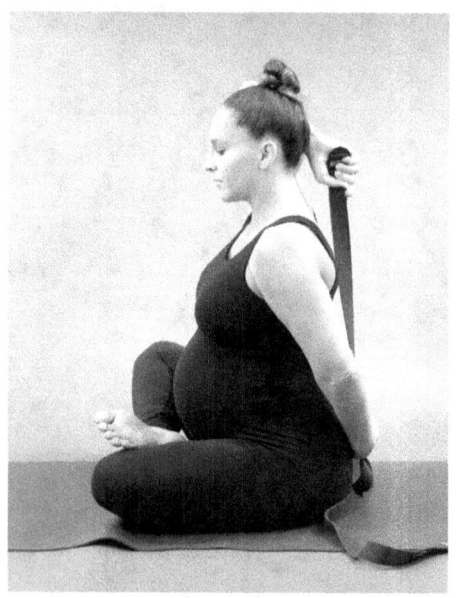

The Cow Face pose is an excellent way to open the chest and hips, and stretch the shoulders and ankles. These effects are very beneficial during pregnancy, since they help you breathe easier, and release any tension and pain in your hips. You may need to place a towel or other padding under your hips and spine as you perform this pose to make sure you remain aligned and don't compress your stomach by hunching over.

How To Do It

- Position your legs so that the left foot is by the right hip, and the right foot is by the left hip, or as close to this position that your belly will allow. Go just far enough to feel the stretch in your hips, but not farther.

- Sit up straight, and stack the knees by placing the left knee directly on top of the right knee if you can.

- Holding onto a strap or towel, bring your right arm up toward the ceiling, bending your elbow so that your hand falls to the center of your back, and the strap is allowed to dangle freely.

- Hold your left arm out to the side, and bend the elbow so that your hand is going up the center of your back, take hold of the strap, and inch your hands as close together as is comfortable for the greatest stretch.

- Sit up straight and bring both elbows in toward your body. Hold this position, taking several deep breaths here.

- Come back to the center, and reposition so you can complete the pose with the other leg on top.

Things to Remember

Your joints are much more relaxed during pregnancy, especially in the hips. Rather than pushing as far as possible, keep the stretches gentle to avoid over-stretching.

DOWNWARD DOG MODIFIED FOR PREGNANCY

The standard Downward Dog strengthens the arms and shoulders, eases stiffness and pain in the upper back, and boosts circulation. This pose can be dangerous during pregnancy, due to the positioning of the belly above the heart. Because of this, it is recommended that pregnant women perform only a modified Downward Dog, which is more of a supported forward bend.

How To Do It

You will need a straight-backed chair to perform the modified form. Make sure it's placed flat against a wall or other stable surface to keep in place.

- Stretch your arms out from the shoulders in front of you, placing your hands on the back of the chair.

- Slowly walk your feet backwards until your back and arms are parallel to the floor. Make sure that your knees are straight, and that your legs are directly in line with your hips, and your feet parallel.

- Maintain your head position so that it is in line with your spine, rather than hanging.

- Breathe in deeply through the nose and slowly exhale. Hold the posture for three to five breaths.

- Inhale deeply, and walk your feet back in toward

the chair, exhaling as you return to the starting position.

Things to Remember

When performing this or any other pose that requires additional support during pregnancy, make sure you are using something that is stable, and will remain in one place throughout the movements.

Again, your joints are considerably looser during pregnancy, so don't force the stretch too far. Listen to your body, and stop if anything feels uncomfortable.

HIP CIRCLES AND PELVIC FLOOR LIFTS

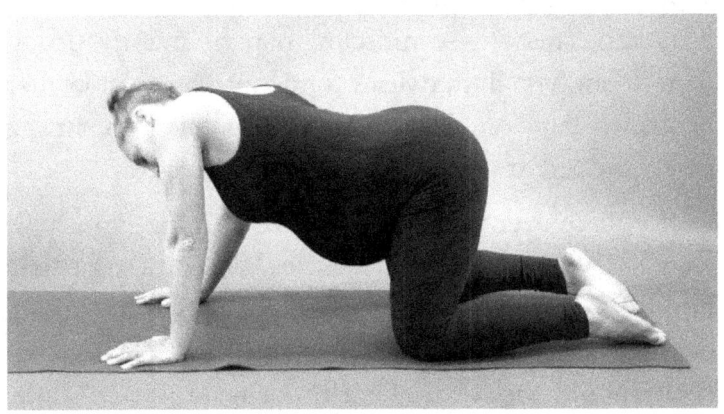

Hip circles help to loosen the hips and lower back, relieving pain and stiffness. They also help the baby to move into a better position for the upcoming labor by creating more space in your hips.

How To Do It

You will start the hip circles in the Cat pose, but feel free to widen your knees just a bit to make the move more comfortable. While in the Cat pose, start moving your hips, following an imaginary figure "8". You can keep your movements small, or make them larger, or even do a combination of the two – just listen to your body, and do what feels best.

Pelvic Floor Lifting

The pelvic floor muscles are the group of muscles holding up your pelvic organs. These muscles are important for maintaining urinary and bowel continence, but during your pregnancy they must also support the additional weight of your uterus and baby. This can cause these muscles to permanently droop or weaken, which may lead to incontinence and other problems later on. To remedy this, pelvic floor lifting can be added at the end of your hip circles.

If you've ever stopped the flow of urine, you have engaged your pelvic floor muscles. When doing pelvic floor lifts, you will focus on three stages. Start by taking deep breath in. As you exhale, lift your pelvic floor (you should feel a drawing up sensation). Continue your exhale, contracting your pelvic floor again and lower abdomen. Do this one more time as you exhale. Do not hold your breath at the end of the exhale, but immediately relax you pelvic floor muscles and start the inhale. As you take your next inhale, completely release your pelvic floor contraction. Repeat this process, focusing on the stages as you lift and let go of the contraction, to help improve the overall strength of these muscles.

If you find it difficult to coordinate the contraction with the breathing, you can hold continuously for the entire exhale, counting "One, hold, hold, hold. Two, hold, hold, hold. Three, hold, hold, hold."

PIGEON POSE

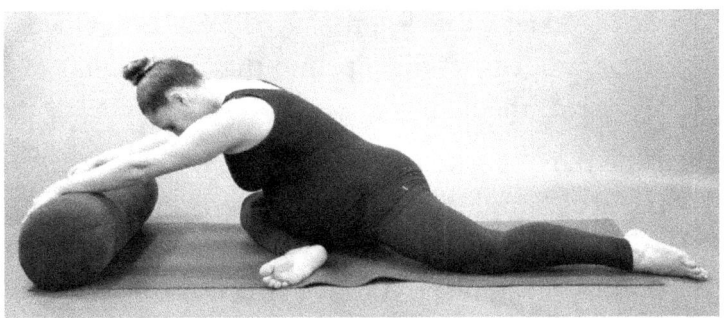

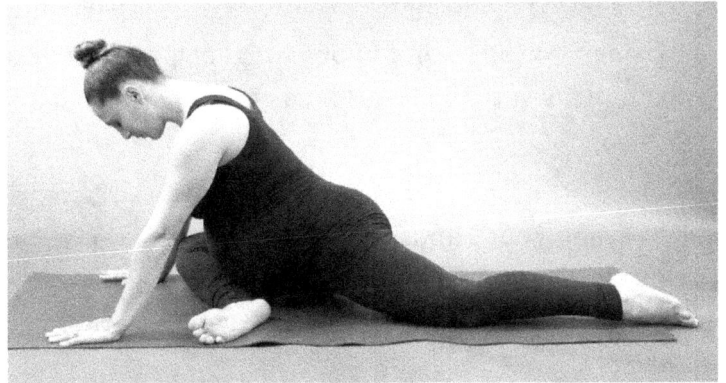

The Pigeon pose is great for those in their third trimester, since it helps to relieve the sciatic pain caused when the baby puts pressure on your nerves. Pigeon also opens the hips, and releases the tension that builds up in your lower back.

How To Do It

During pregnancy, especially as your belly grows, you will likely need to incorporate a pillow or use your arms to create a pillow for your head.

- Start on all fours in the tabletop position.

- Slowly extend one leg, making sure it's stretched straight out from the hip, and that the thigh is level with the floor.

- Slide the opposite leg to the front, making sure the heel is in line with the opposite hip, and that the knee is directly behind your arm on the same side. You can place your leg either in front of your belly, or behind it for a less intense stretch.

- Using your arms, hold your weight up so that you can make sure that your hips are in line with each other.

- Once positioned properly, sink into the stretch by using your hands to walk your upper body out until your chest is over the front thigh. While moving into the position, inhale slowly and deeply.

- Hold the stretch for as long as possible, making sure to inhale and exhale deeply throughout the hold.

- To raise yourself back to the starting position, walk your hands slowly back towards your hips until you are back in the upright position.

- Lean your body in the direction of the leg in front, and bring the back leg around so you are in a sitting position.

- Repeat on both sides.

If you feel any pain performing this pose, slowly ease out of it, back into the sitting position, and try again another day.

HIP OPENERS

Prenatal hip openers provide relief from tightness, and help prepare your body for delivery. The following are some of the best hip opener yoga poses that help do both of these things and relieve stress.

Seated Hip Opener

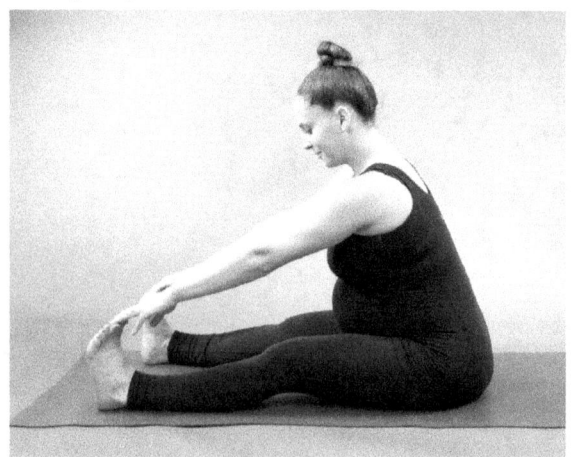

How To Do It

In this pose, which is a modified Forward Fold, take care not to compress your belly.

- Sit with your legs extended in front of you, your spine lengthened and tall.

- Reach forward to grab your toes. If your belly is large enough to be compressed by this, use a towel or belt and wrap it around the soles of your feet and bend forward only as much as is comfortable.

While doing this breathe deeply for five to ten breaths, exhaling as you come back to the starting position on the last one.

Alternate Seated Hip Opener

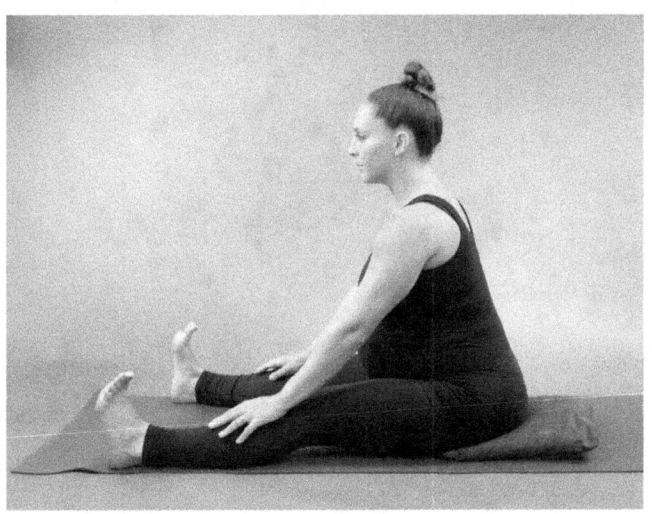

How To Do It

- Fold up a towel and place it under your hips and tailbone, or use a small pillow, so that your pelvis is slightly tilted, making it easier for you to lean forward.

As in earlier poses, take care not to hunch over and compress your belly.

COBBLER'S POSE

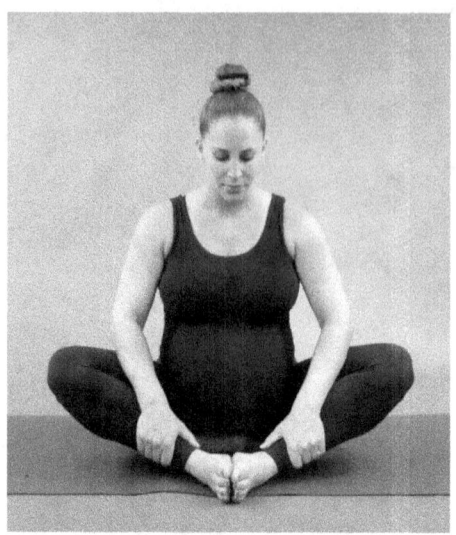

This hip opener should be done with care, making sure not to pull your feet in too far.

How To Do It

- Sit with legs extended in front of you, then bend the knees until the soles of your feet touch.

- Pull the feet toward your body as much as feel comfortable without scrunching down onto your belly.

- Hold onto the inside of your feet, so that your elbows are on your calves.

- Lean forward slightly with a straight back, making sure you don't compress your belly, breathe deeply for four to six breaths, and return to the starting position.

WINDSHIELD WIPERS

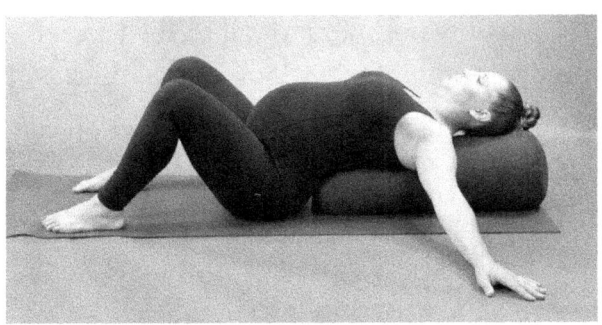

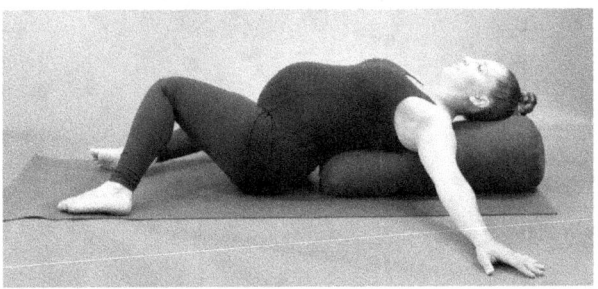

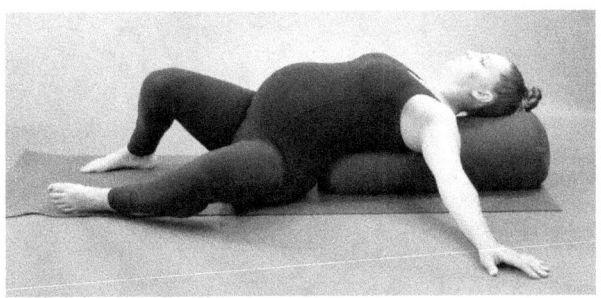

How To Do It

- Lie on your back with a towel or blanket under your upper back.

- Bend your knees and position your legs so your feet are wider than your hips, and stretch your

63

arms out in a T-shape to the sides.

- Slowly allow both legs to fall to the left, while you move your head to look to the right.

- Bring knees back to center and repeat on right side.

When doing this pose, make sure breathe deeply, and do the pose four to six times on both sides, dropping your knees only as far to each side as feels comfortable.

CHAIR POSE

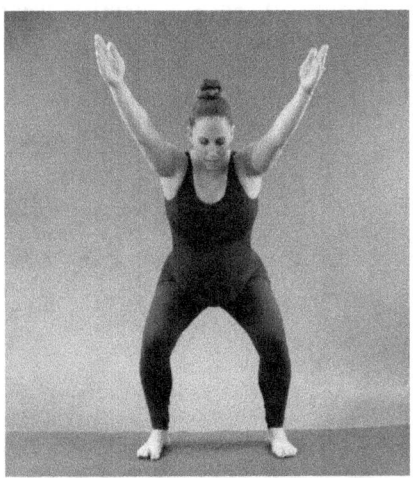

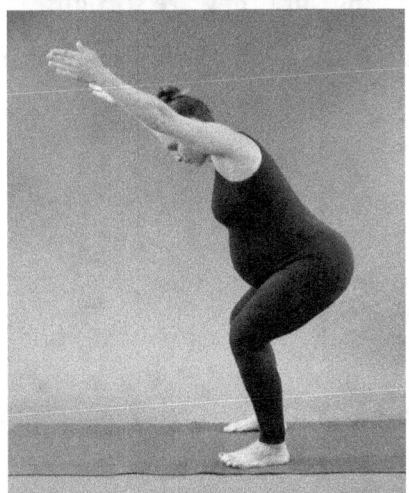

The Chair pose strengthens the entire lower body, ankles to thighs, as well as the hips, buttocks, and back. It's also a great pose for stretching the shoulders and Achilles tendons, opening the chest to make breathing easier, and helping to tone and strengthen the heart. Despite all these benefits, it is not a difficult pose—it's actually considered a beginner pose, although it can be incorporated into more challenging once, and is often used as a transitional move.

How To Do It

You will begin this posture in the Mountain pose. If you're more advanced, feel free to stand with your feet together, but for beginners and heavily pregnant women, it's recommended to keep your feet at hip width or wider to provide a more stable base.

- Inhale, then slowly raise your arms over your head, making sure they are straight.

- Exhale and bend your knees until your thighs are parallel to the floor. If you are unable to, simply go as low as you can.

- As you lower yourself, your torso will form a near right angle with your thighs, and your knees will move slightly past your feet.

- Push your elbows back towards your ears, while drawing your shoulder blades in towards your back. Make sure your ribcage does not move forward, and pull your tailbone down, making sure to keep your back in a long line.

- Make sure you're shifting your weight onto your heels. Your toes should not be pressed into the floor.

- Hold the pose, making sure to breathe deeply the entire time.
- When coming out of the pose, inhale and straighten yourself with your legs, lifting yourself through your arms.

MODIFIED SUN SALUTATION

Some yoga moves should only be performed during pregnancy if they've been modified, including Sun Salutations. The modified version of this pose removes the Upward Dog Pose, which can cause the placenta to tear and too much pressure on your belly.

Note: if you find coordinating the inhaling and exhaling with each movement difficult, don't worry about it too much, just do one or the other with every movement. The important part is that you keep breathing to infuse your body and mind with loads of fresh oxygen.

How To Do It

- Begin with your feet spread to hip width. Hands in front of your heart, palms touching. (Anjali mudra)

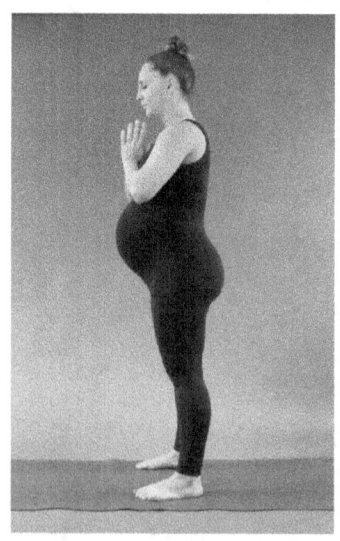

- Inhale, sweeping your arms up. If you want more of a stretch along the front of your body, tighten up your hips and thighs and lean back slightly.

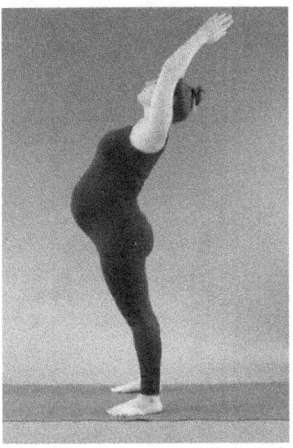

- Exhale slowly and fold yourself forward, making sure to keep your breastbone lifted to prevent putting pressure on your belly. Place your hands on your thighs or knees, whichever is more comfortable.

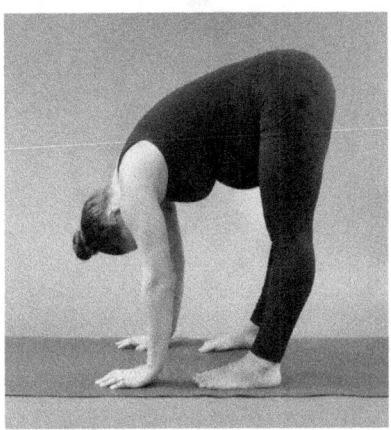

- Inhale, looking straight ahead to stretch the spine.

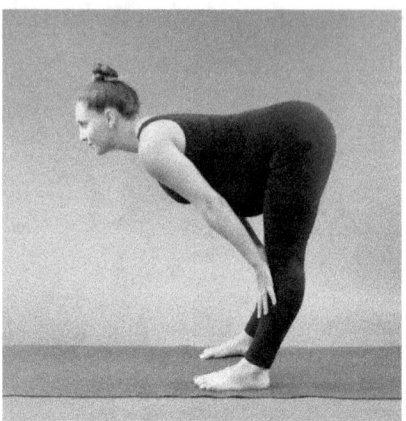

- Exhale, placing your hands on the floor or on your yoga blocks if needed. Bend your knees as much as necessary to get your hands to the floor.

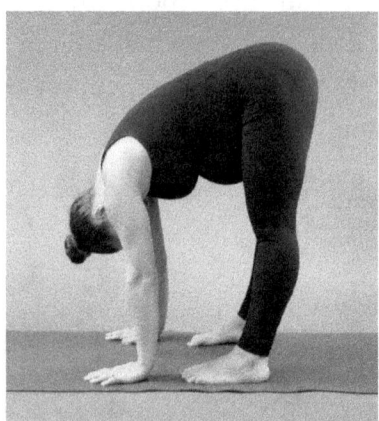

- Inhale, step the right leg back, then the left, and come into modified plank pose, weight on your knees, with your feet up.

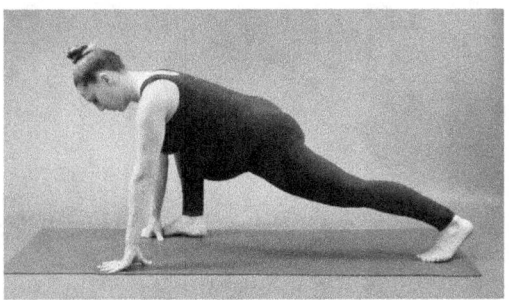

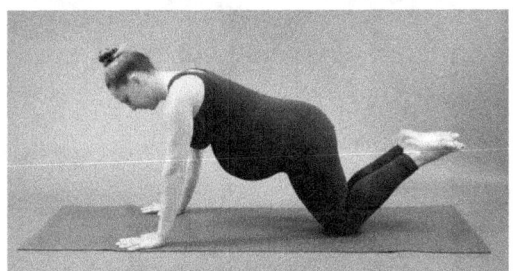

- Exhale, shift your weight back to Child's Pose, toes tucked under, buttocks resting on heels, with your arms straight out in front of you.

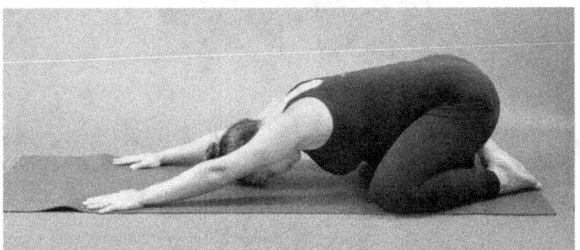

- Inhale, rock the body forward again to modified plank position.

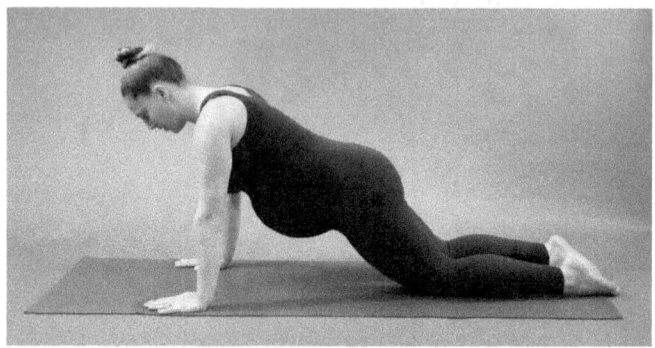

- Exhale, maintaining modified plank pose, curl your toes under.
- Bring your left foot up to meet your hands, then your right foot.

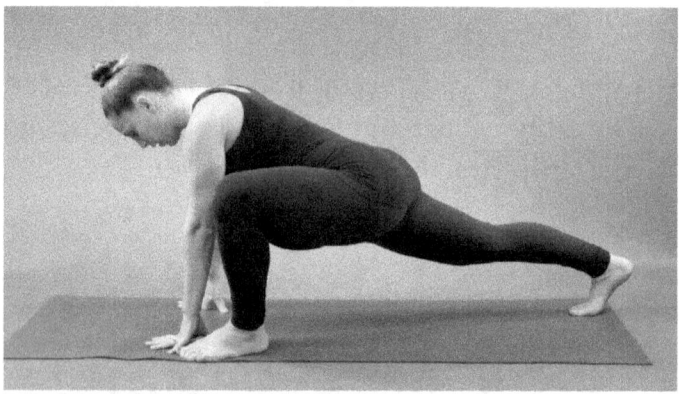

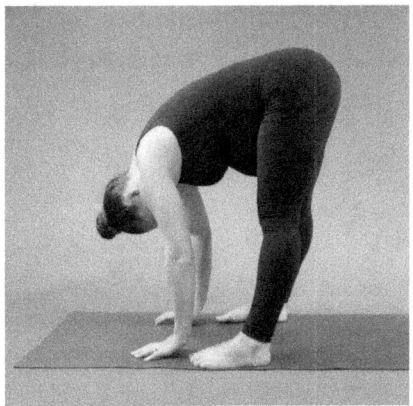

- Inhale, forward bend.
- Exhale, lift your body to starting position.

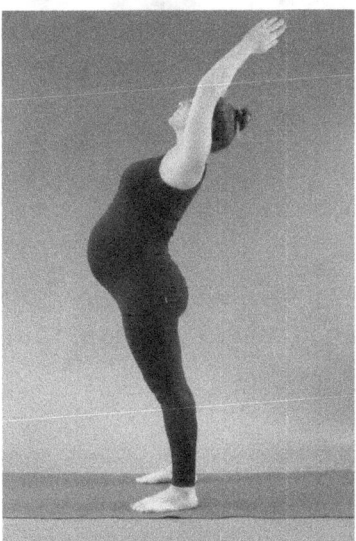

- Slowly inhale, stretching your arms up toward the sky. Lean back if it feels good to you, be careful how far you go and don't compress your lower back. If you do lean backward, think of lifting your chest as you lean your arms back.

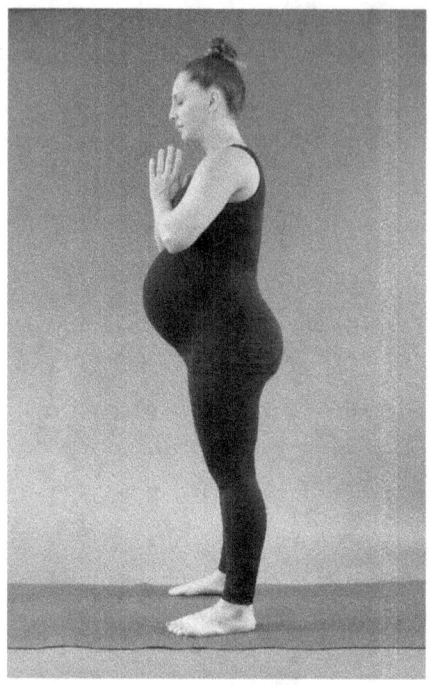

- Exhale, bringing your hands back in front of your heart in Anjali mudra position, palms touching.

MOUNTAIN POSE

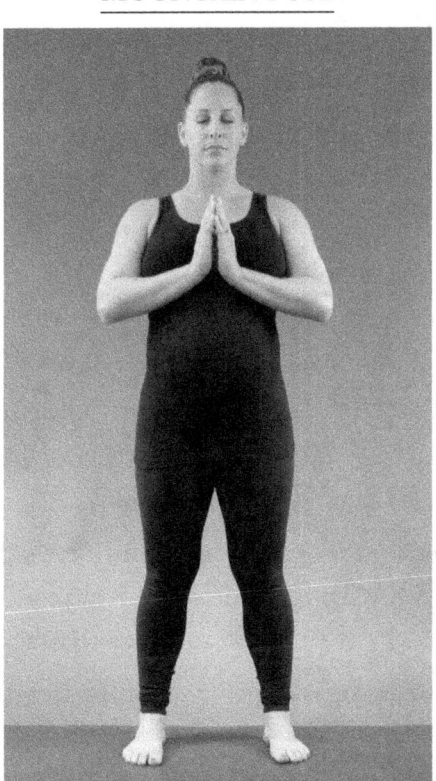

The Mountain pose, or *tadasana*, strengthens and centers the body, which makes it great for when your hormones flare, or when you simply need a moment to focus. This pose can be done at the beginning of your postures, in the middle, or any time you need catch your breath.

How To Do It

- Stand with your feet in a position that is hip

width apart, with the outside line of your feet parallel – your toes may be pointed in slightly to achieve this position.

- Stand up straight, with your pelvis tucked in slightly so that you feel just a bit of engagement in your core.

- Push your shoulders down and back so that your chest is open, and align your head so that your chin is parallel to the floor and in a straight line with your back.

- Reach up through the crown of your head toward the sky. This elongates the spine.

- You can do this pose with your hands down at your sides with the palms in, or you can reach towards the sky to add more challenge.

- Hold the position for 30 seconds, breathing deeply.

Things to Remember

While performing the pose, focus on deep inhalations and exhalations, paying attention to the way in which the air enters and exits your body. You can take advantage of this position even further by focusing the cleansing, healing breaths directly to areas that are tired or sore.

This is a usually a very safe pose during pregnancy, but if you do notice any discomfort, bring yourself out of the pose slowly and rest. If there is too much tension in your lower back, allow your knees to bend slightly to relieve it, slowly working your way to holding the pose without the need to modify it.

HORSE POSE

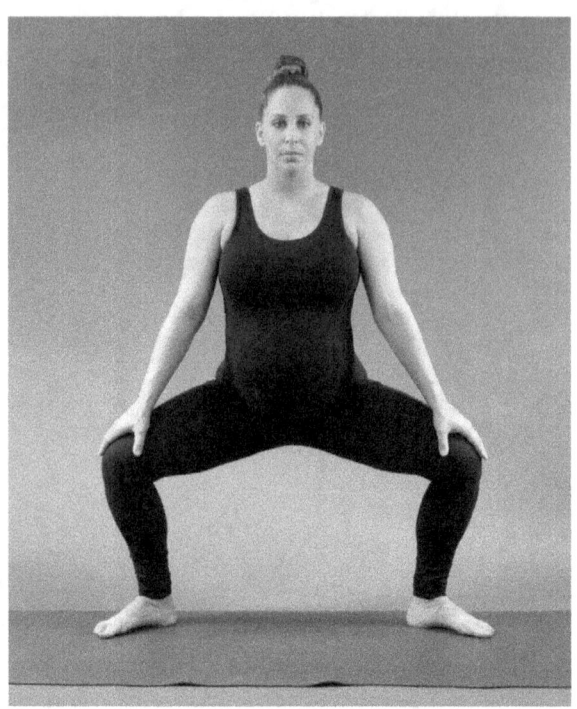

The Horse pose stabilizes and strengthens the muscles in the inner thighs, hips, and pelvis, which is especially important for pregnant women. But it also works the quads, calves, shins, and arches of the feet, helping to create a strong stable base that will be beneficial as you move into the later stages of your pregnancy, when balance becomes more important— and more difficult.

How To Do It

The Horse pose is another posture that needs to be

modified during pregnancy to provide extra stability. This can either be with the hands on the knees, or you can perform the pose with your back against the wall for support if necessary.

- Stand with your feet at a wider position than your hips, and with your feet turned so that they are facing 10 and 2 o'clock.

- Slowly bend your knees and slide down, keeping your knees and ankles in line, and over the second toe. Slide down approximately six inches so that your thighs are getting close to parallel to the floor, making sure to practice deep breathing, with slow inhales and exhales while holding the position.

Things to Remember

When doing this pose, keep your pelvis square, with your spine drawn down toward the floor. Your pelvis should not be tilted forward or backward. If you're having problems with this, place your hands at your hips to feel the correct alignment.

If this variation of the Horse pose is too challenging or causes pain, move your feet in closer so that your stance is not as wide. You will slowly loosen the hips over time, allowing you to use the wider stance. You can also lessen the intensity by not lowering yourself as deeply.

TREE POSE

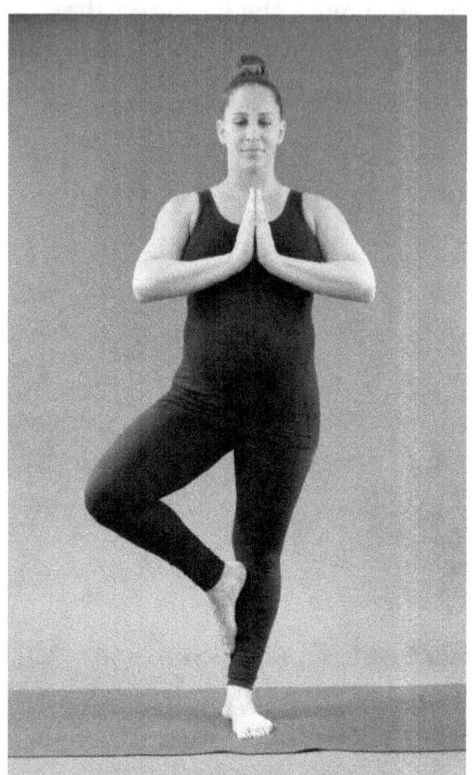

The Tree pose is used as a balancing posture, which can help maintain coordination as you move through your pregnancy. It also gives you time to concentrate on your body and breathing deeply to get the greatest benefit from the pose.

How To Do It

Many women have difficulty balancing as they progress in their pregnancies, as baby weight increases and your center of balance shifts. Because of this, it's recommended you perform the Tree pose near a wall or use a chair for additional support.

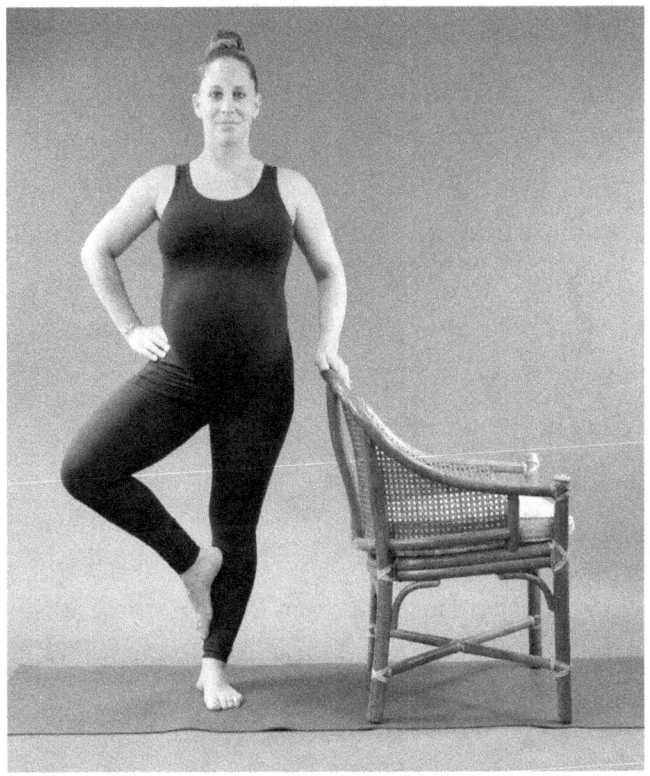

- Stand with your feet together on your mat, with your arms at your sides. While in this position, shift backwards and forwards slightly to find your center of balance.
- Once you've found your balance, focus on feeling the grounding of your legs into the earth.

- Focus on a single point in front you, slowly raising one foot along the inside of the other leg. Move the bottom of that foot to any point along your calf or up to the inner thigh, making sure not to stop at the knee.

- Tighten the standing leg, and feel both legs working together to balance you in the position.

- You can either bring your arms completely over-head, or bring them to your chest with the palms together.

- Release the pose slowly, continuing to breathe deeply as you lower your foot.

- Repeat the pose on the opposite leg.

You may need to relax the pose a bit as your joints loosen during pregnancy. If you have trouble main-taining the this pose, simply keep your foot at the calf level or lower, ensure that you don't become unstable and fall. And, if needed, use that nearby wall for balance.

WIDE STRADDLE FORWARD BEND

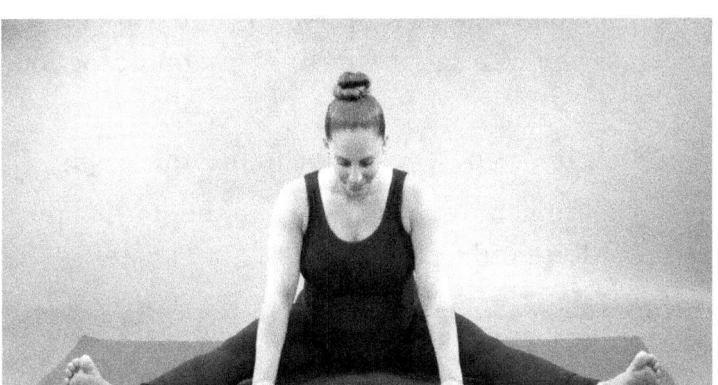

The Wide Straddle Forward Bend stretches your back, legs and arms, and improves circulation to the upper body. This is a calming pose, and beneficial during pregnancy. However, it's not recommended for women who are in their third trimester—always make sure to speak with your doctor before doing this and other yoga poses.

How To Do It

- Sit with your legs as wide apart as possible, toes facing up.

- Inhale deeply, press your palms onto the mat in front of your belly.

- Start to bend your elbows to bring your chest as close to the mat as your belly will allow.

- Rest your elbows on the floor, or a block.

- Drop your head down between your arms, or cross your arms to use them as a support for your head.

- While in this pose, continue to breathe deeply.

- Exhale and move slowly back to the starting position. Repeat the pose twice.

Things to Remember

If your thighs feel very tight, you can bend your knees slightly. Keep your back in a straight line throughout the movements; it should not be rounded when you reach the final position.

LEGS UP THE WALL CHAIR VERSION

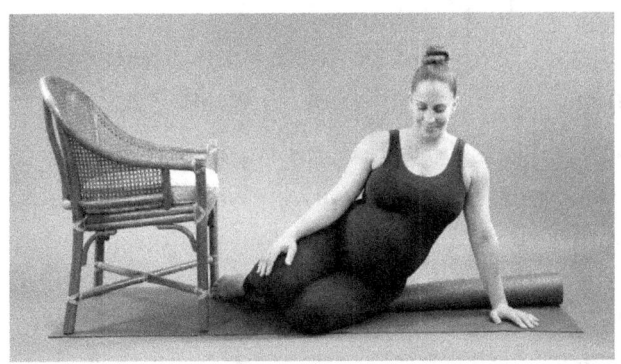

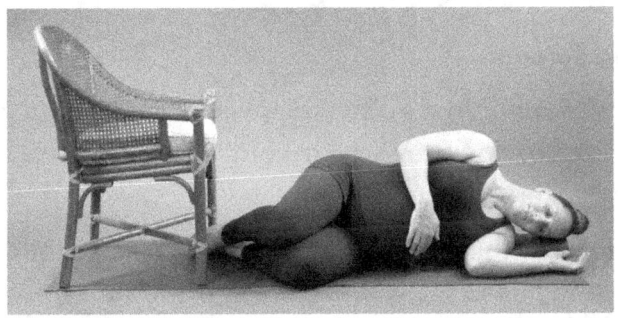

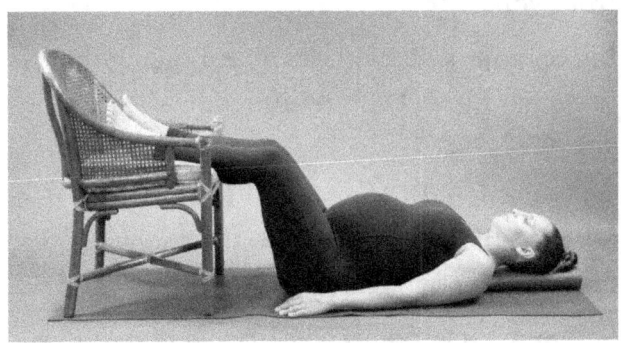

The Legs up the Wall pose is a restorative inversion pose that aids blood and lymph circulation, eases back pain, assists with insomnia, improves digestion, posture and more.

This pose should be used with care for pregnant women, and not at all after 36 weeks.

The pose is very restorative, but awkward to get into as your pregnancy progresses. Here is the chair variation that can be used during this time. Depending on the length of your legs, you may need to add padding to the chair so that your knees can be near a 90-degree angle.

How To Do It

You will need a bolster, blanket or a rolled up yoga mat to provide support for your back and keep your body slightly elevated.

- Place a chair at the end of your mat, up against something that will prevent it from sliding away from you.

- Lie on your side, with your seat facing the chair, and your knees bent, pointing away from the chair.

- As you roll onto your back onto the bolster or blanket, lift one leg up onto the chair seat, then lift the other leg up.

- Situate yourself on the bolster so that your hips are gently sloping down from your back, and your back is elevated.

- Lie back, relax and breathe deeply for 3 to 5 minutes.

- Come out of the pose in reverse order, bringing one leg down to the floor, then turning your body, bringing the other leg down, and lie on your side.

- Bring your hands underneath your shoulders, and push up to sitting.

CORPSE POSE

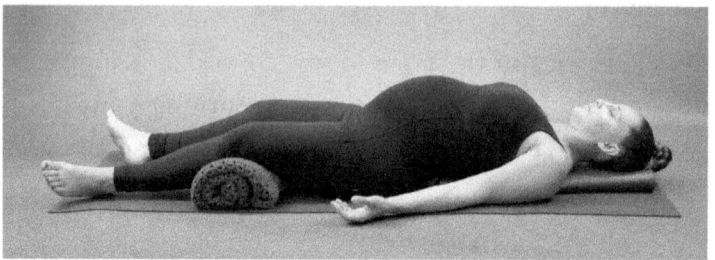

Corpse pose or Savasana, is the ultimate pose for relaxation, which is why it is typically done at the end of your yoga practice. It will allow you to take a few moments to enjoy the inner peace you've created, and allow you to relax after you've completed the poses. Savasana allows you to embody all the benefits of your practice, utilizing the additional oxygen and circulation of fresh blood and nutrients to your own organs and your fetus'.

Most yoga practices end with several minutes spent in this pose, and it can easily be the most calming part of the whole session. The pose puts the body totally at ease by emphasizing complete relaxation. Corpse pose triggers the body's "relaxation response," a state of deep rest that slows the breathing and lowers the blood pressure while quieting the nervous system. It is the ideal way to finish your practice because, in this relaxed yoga pose, you simply lie back and practice letting go.

How To Do It

You will need to make some modifications when doing the Corpse pose while pregnant, as it is not recommend to spend too much time on your back. During the first and second trimesters, however, all you need to do is add pillows beneath your head and under the curve of your spine. As you progress in your pregnancy, add props as necessary.

Have your rolled up mat, bolster, blocks or blankets available, so you can experiment with what feels best to you at any given stage.

- Start seated on the mat with your legs bent and feet flat on the floor. Inhale deeply and then exhale, leaning back onto your forearms and slightly lifting your pelvis off the mat. Place the sacrum flat on the mat by tucking the tailbone toward the foot of the mat. Deeply inhale and slowly extend one leg, then the other, as you soften the groin and turn the feet slightly outward. Exhale deeply as you soften your lower back and feel your body sink gently onto the mat.

- Inhaling, use your hands to lift the base of your skull away from your neck as you soften the muscles in the back of the neck. Exhale deeply as you broaden the base of your skull and wiggle your body around a bit to ensure that it feels symmetrical on the mat.

- Deeply inhale and reach both arms toward the ceiling as you rock your body slightly side to side to broaden your back against the mat. Deeply exhale and release your arms to the mat, turning the thumbs slightly outward and resting the backs of the hands on the mat.

- Deeply inhale and then exhale while you concentrate on softening your tongue, your facial muscles, your scalp, and the skin on your forehead. Close your eyes and let them sink back into your skull; allow your brain to settle and do the same.

- For the first minute or so, focus on your breathing. Breathe deeply and slowly, being mindful of each inhalation and exhalation. Deeply inhale, then completely relax and let the exhale flow out. Extend your exhalations by a second or two, making them longer than your inhalations. Inhale deeply and breathe with your whole body, feeling the breath move the belly, and slightly rock the hips, shoulders, and spine. Feel the breath filter through every muscle and organ in your body, calming and soothing every cell.

- Take this moment to connect with your unborn child, appreciating yourself for taking such good care of the two of you, infusing the fetus with oxygen, fresh blood supply and nutrients.

Visualize your baby smiling and happy.

- Now just begin to let go. Do not focus on the breath; allow it to become soft and natural, and simply observe where it goes. Let yourself relax completely. If you have time constraints, you may want to set an alarm in case you drift off.

Things to Remember

If you experience any discomfort—even with the pillows—try placing a rolled towel under you knees. If you are in your third trimester, you will need to do a modified *Savasana* lying on your left side. Use the pillows that would go under your back, and place them under your right knee, bringing it over your left. This will allow you to enjoy the relaxation without placing dangerous pressure on the vena cava, which runs along your right side. Breathe deep, and stay in the position for five to fifteen minutes.

Conclusion

Since this is such an amazing and special time in your life, you will want to spend some time meditating on what it means to be able to bring a new life into the world, and the special bond that you and your child will share forever. Not only are you creating this new life from your own body, you are passing down your and your baby's fathers' inherent genetic strengths.

The time will zoom by, and before you know it, you'll have a baby in your life that will need a lot of care and attention. Try to avoid getting caught up in all the hubbub that expectant motherhood entails—baby showers, choosing a name, shopping for strollers and furniture, and getting your work situation taken care of for maternity leave. These things are important of course, but just as importantly, your Easy Yoga practice will allow you to set aside time to care of yourself, stay calm, and nurture yourself and your baby. Your Easy Yoga practice may be the last time you get to spend in reflection for a while, and you can treat it as a special time when you communicate to the growing child within you.

There will be some days that you might just feel too tired to get on the mat, and do any postures, and on those days, simply being mindful and doing your deep breathing will be great for you. Because with yoga, you are not only doing postures, you are becoming more conscious of yourself, including the life inside you.

Since your pregnancy can be stressful at times, here are a series of affirmations that you can use to center and calm yourself any time you need to.

Affirmations for Expectant Mothers

I accept and welcome the life growing inside me.

All of my emotions exist to benefit me and I allow them to wash over me without judgment.

I accept my body, with all the variations of sensation that are happening.

I delight in the gift of life that I possess and can share.

My body is a source of nurturing to my baby and me.

My body knows what to do to give birth perfectly to a perfect child.

I am learning to go with the flow, I am letting go of my need to control.

I feel immense gratitude for the power of my breath to heal and soothe me.

Energy is always flowing, and I can relax with any discomfort, knowing it will soon pass.

I am grateful for the support of those around me.

My body is surrounded with white light and healing energy, including my baby.

I am made from the same stuff as the stars. I am magnificent.

Acknowledgements

I wish to thank everyone who helped make this book possible:

- My loving husband, Michael Garver, who patiently supports all my creative endeavors, and who shot the photos for this book.

- Samantha Harte, my beautiful, "ready-to-pop" model.

- My eagle-eyed editor, Sarah Jacobs.

- My good-humored and thorough researcher, Ryn Gargulinski.

About Patricia Bacall

Patricia Bacall is an internationally acknowledged authority in the field of personal growth, and teaches individuals and group classes throughout the world on how to live happier, more fulfilling and creative lives, attracting people of all backgrounds and ages.

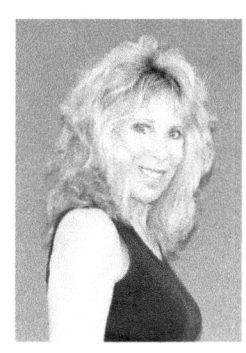

As a personal coach and workshop leader, Patricia has a practical approach that is both engaging and intuitive. She is known for her ability to resonate with people and empower them to live freer and more satisfying lives. Participants often comment on her clarity of communication and thorough knowledge of her subject matter.

With her gentle and positive approach, she assists in healing by first teaching people to love and appreciate themselves as strong and unique individuals, and then giving them the tools they need to achieve their dreams and goals.

Patricia's journey began in 1980 as a personal trainer, teaching people how to improve their fitness, health and wellbeing. Realizing the importance of the mind-body connection and the healing benefits of yoga, she received certifications as a yoga instructor and massage therapist.

During the late '80s, Patricia learned the Vivation breathwork technique, which helps people create resolution of their most negative emotions using a simple yet exceptionally powerful process. Working extensively with Jim Leonard, the founder of Vivation®, she became one of the best-trained breathwork professionals in the United States. Patricia uses the Vivation technique in her workshops and practice to "supercharge" the healing process by uncovering and resolving suppressed emotions.

To round out her education in body, mind and spirit wellness, Patricia has extensively studied yoga, Pilates, and massage, and holds several credentials in these disciplines. She serves on the board of the Associated Vivation Professionals in the United States and is a contributor to personal health publications and websites on the subjects of emotional overeating, physical vitality, overcoming emotional negativity, energy work and yoga.

To My Readers:

Thank you for buying and reading this book.

If you enjoyed it, please leave a review. Your review is important because it helps others make educated buying choices, and allows us to continue to bring you the kind of valuable books and resources that make your life better.

To see our library of books to make your life better, visit:
www.benesserrapub.com